THE HEALTHY WAY

Finding the Power to Create a Healthier Mind and Body

By Dr. Ann B. Davis

Naturopathic Doctor
Licensed Massage Therapist

Table of Contents

About the Author

Dr. Ann B. Davis is a native Texan very happy to be back in her beloved Texas.

Dr. Davis graduated from Austin School of Massage Therapy in Austin, Texas and obtained her Naturopathic Doctor degree from Westbrook University in New Mexico while continuing to pursue her corporate career. She is now dispensing counsel and encouragement to clients on nutrition, detoxification, and raw foods. Go to **http://www.DrAnnBDavis.com** to learn more about her services. She not only coaches and teaches in her local area but holds teleclasses and telephone consultations with people all over the world.

Chapter 1
What's In It for Me?

I enjoyed all my studies of natural health and healing but the information that really fired my interest and passion didn't come until my very last class. I actually had thought I was finished then discovered I needed three more credits. There was a brand new class that had just become available and it was on the subject of raw foods. Not raw meat but raw fruits, vegetables, nuts and seeds. It sounded intriguing so I signed up for it.

The first book I read was "How I Conquered Cancer Naturally" by Eydie Mae Hunsberger. I was fascinated from the very beginning. She told her story about finding the lump in her breast, exploring mainstream medical options then rejecting them, then hearing about natural means of healing and meeting someone who pointed her in the right direction. She ended up spending two weeks at Ann Wigmore's Hippocrates Health Institute in Boston (this was in the 1970s) then went home to make 100% raw vegan eating her way of life. She was healed of her cancer and discovered that straying off her food path caused her cancer to start growing again so she stayed on raw food the rest of her life.

I was so astounded to discover something so simple. Giving your body high quality food enables it to heal itself. Our bodies know what to do but they can only operate in a substandard manner when we feed them junk. I was so excited that after reading all the books required for the course I continued to devour everything I could find about the raw food way of living.

This was in the late 1990's and there wasn't a whole lot available then about it. Most of the people who promoted it were a bit strange in many ways. Now it's more mainstream but still looked at askance by some.

As I continued to learn about it I encountered so many testimonials about how people's bodies healed after changing their diet to include more raw food. I wanted what they had. I didn't have any major illnesses but I wanted to stay healthy and have more energy. Some of the people I read about were suffering from life-threatening diseases and many of them had multiple illnesses.

Over the years I have added more and more nutritious food to my daily diet but noticed that I still struggled with cravings for comfort foods that were unhealthy. This turned out to be a lot more difficult and I realized that it was about more than just controlling my food. My mental, emotional and spiritual health had to be addressed. So that started another whole area of study which will be ongoing as long as I'm alive. We cannot just work on a part of ourselves, we have to develop all aspects of our beings. The benefits from that have been tremendous because I used to be a very negative person. I have had to detoxify not just my body but my thoughts and feelings also. I'm still working on it and discovering new things every day. It's an exciting journey.

The purpose of this book is to get you started. I didn't want to overwhelm you with too much information because that can be paralyzing. Just pretend you're in kindergarten or first grade and you're learning the alphabet. Most people don't realize that they have any control over what happens in their lives or what thoughts or feelings they experience. They passively let negative circumstances poison their thoughts, feelings, relationships, careers, health, etc. I'm here to tell you that you do have control and you do have a choice. All you have to do is learn what to do and put it into action. Fasten your seatbelt and let's go for a ride!

Chapter 2
Who is Ann B. Davis?

A healthy body is more important than a thin, beautiful body. I just want to make that clear. I am not advocating a model-thin body or perfection that is unobtainable. But we are surrounded with toxic food choices everywhere we go – supermarkets, restaurants, and home kitchens. These food choices not only fail to provide nourishment but many times they are also addictive and our body screams for more in an attempt to get what it needs to survive. My goal is to educate you and help you make healthy food and lifestyle choices for the purpose of optimum health. When you are healthy and fit you are able to give your time and attention to the activities and people that matter most to you instead of being constantly badgered by cravings and self-bashing. I invite you to clear your mind of all the diet plans and attempts at controlling your food and join me in getting down to basics. Let's just keep it simple!

I easily stayed slender during the first part of my life. Whenever I gained a few pounds I'd go on a diet and get back to my desired weight within a short period of time. But then in my late 30s major events started happening in my life and I began to unravel. I realized that all the ways I'd coped and dealt with things in the past just weren't working and I couldn't keep making the same mistakes with relationships, jobs, etc. So I started on my personal growth journey but turned to food for comfort. My weight started inching upward and dieting was no longer easy and quick. For the first time I couldn't seem to stay on a diet for more than a day or two. Sometimes I would manage to lose about eight pounds then it would creep back on again. As my 40s turned into my 50s I began to despair and hate myself even more. I just couldn't seem to get my act together.

Then in my 50s I lost my career in the midst of an economic downturn. I promptly plunged into the basement of despair. I had been studying naturopathy for several years prior to this so decided to make a new career of nutrition counseling and helping people get healthy. I opened an herb shop which was a disaster financially then after closing it I tried to get a private practice going. That didn't go much of anywhere either. I learned a great deal from these experiences but I was in an even bigger mess financially and still thirty pounds overweight. That may not seem huge to some people but it was enormous to me. I was embarrassed about not even being able to follow my own advice. I ate a pretty healthy diet but too much of a good thing is still fattening.

I finally hit the bottom in the fall of 2006. I had tried everything I could think of to turn my situation around and had only succeeded in making it worse. I knew that I was inclined to negativity and depression and had improved some but nowhere near enough to help me see any light at the end of the tunnel. One morning when I was talking to God (whining is a better description) a Bible verse came to my remembrance. "Seek first His kingdom and His righteousness, and all these things will be given to you as well" (Matthew 6:33, NIV). I wondered what would happen if I did that. Just put everything else aside, stop trying to find a solution, and spend hours every day seeking God. I made a decision right then and there to do that. I am an early riser and I would get up, make myself a pot of tea and go upstairs to my office and study the Word, listen to teachings by people I respected and write in my journal. I already had many books, tapes and CDs at my disposal but I ordered more, especially anything having to do with prosperity. I also read books about abundance, success, positive thinking, manifesting, etc. by many different authors. I trusted the Holy Spirit to let me know if any particular book or belief wasn't for me. Some of them I tossed after reading them a little bit and others I have read over and over, underlining on every page.

Within two weeks our financial situation started improving. I was delighted about that but my seeking God had turned into a real search for Him and I so much enjoyed my mornings of study. It was no longer just about the money. I saw that God wants us to be prosperous in all areas of our lives and I was determined to learn more and see what great purposes and plans He had for me. I was beginning to see that He was not the big bad guy in the sky looking to rap me over the head anytime I did something wrong. He loves me and wants the very best for me.

The next thing I discovered was writing. I had kept journals for years and had found them helpful but this was a different kind of writing. Right before Christmas a friend loaned me "Write It Down, Make It Happen" by Henriette Klauser. One of the first things I wrote was that I wanted to move back to Texas by bluebonnet season in 2007. I didn't see any way that could happen. We were living in Colorado in a very bad real estate market. After returning to Colorado from our Christmas Texas trip we had a miserably cold and snowy January and I was so homesick. On top of that our ARM mortgage suddenly went up 3% and we were staggering under our enormous house payment which hadn't been small to begin with. In February I just decided it was time to sell and move back to Texas. My husband had been working from home for awhile and it was now possible for us to live anywhere we wanted and he wanted to go back home also. So we put the house up for sale and I started writing about it. It sold to the first looker for a fair price and things just sped up from there. I wrote about the house we needed to find in our new location and it showed up. I have been writing daily about everything since then.

I continued to read books about abundance, the law of attraction and anything else that looked remotely helpful. I was being drawn more and more to writing and teaching but didn't know yet what it would really look like in reality. I had sensed as far back as 1996 that I was to have a weight loss business/ministry but keep doubting it would ever happen since I still hadn't lost my excess weight. I thought I had to be perfect before I could teach anything. Then it finally dawned on me. My purpose is to be a light-bearer, lighting the path before you. None of the people I have learned from are perfect but something they said or did caused a light bulb to go on in my head and illuminated a new truth for me. I had started this book in 2005 but never finished it because I felt it lacked the key that would enable you to succeed at weight loss or even just changing your food habits for the better. There are already hundreds of books out there about the food aspect of it but very little about how to find the power to make it happen. I gave myself permission to go ahead and made a decision to birth my weight loss business. I've certainly been in labor long enough!

I am now living in my beloved Texas, losing weight and getting fit, and building an exciting health and wellness business. I pray that this book will shed a little light on your path.

By the way, I'm not the Ann B. Davis who played Alice on The Brady Bunch!

Chapter 3
Set Your Mind

First things first. If you don't have control over your thoughts you do not have control over your feelings and actions. You may doubt me but I invite you to do some detective work. A journal is a really key tool because you'll forget the Ah-ha's very quickly. You'll also forget what you ate for breakfast (and what you thought and felt, mentally, emotionally, and physically) by the next day or maybe even by dinner that night. Do you remember what you thought about upon awakening this morning? Was it negative? Did you wish you could go back to sleep and forget about life? Or did you leap out of bed in anticipation of the day and its events? What is going on in your life that contributed to these thoughts? If you had negative thoughts were you able to replace them with positive and go about your business or did the negative thoughts trail after you all day, spawning self-hatred and dissatisfaction with everything and everybody, primarily yourself?

Now you're probably thinking, "I thought she was going to keep it simple!" Well, the food part is simple but humans are complex. This has been the hardest part for me to get. I have tried every diet under the sun. When I was younger they worked easily. But now I can't seem to stay on them. I know the problem is not just the food, it's me and what I'm telling myself about the food and everything else in my life. I've become better at recognizing the lies that I tell myself but I'm still working on being able to deflect them and keep them from harming me. I know that eating pie will not only make me sick but give me extra calories I don't need. I am amazed at how easily I can ignore that lie and stuff some in my mouth as if I believed that it was the most nutritious food on earth.

Most of us have been given food as a reward since childhood. And these were usually the worst kinds of food – sweet, rich, fat laden – with no redeeming qualities except that they made us feel better emotionally, for a few minutes anyway until the guilt started up. In fact, these foods were punishment – punishment to every tissue and cell of our body. Many books have been written about the damage sugar does to our body so I won't go into that here. So we have to change our thinking about what constitutes reward and punishment. We need a whole new set of values where food is concerned! You would think that everyone would value health above certain foods but you will find people making the wrong choices over and over again. Why? What lies are we telling ourselves that goad us into making these choices? This is what you have to find out. Then you have to start changing it.

I can just hear you saying "I've been trying to change it for years!!" Well, me too. But I was going about it all wrong. Have you ever noticed that when you start thinking about something that you don't want to think about that it seems like your brain just gets stuck there and goes on and on and on? You're hungry, tired or frustrated and you just want to pile into a banana split and gorge until you're so full that your brain just shuts down and you feel a little peace? You try not to think about it but your brain just keeps going back to it and creating a whole, huge story around it in vivid color. You can taste, smell and feel it even though it still only exists in your head. How do we stop that process? Once I'm into it I discover that I get very rebellious and don't even want to stop the process. I just want what I want. Well, there are a lot of different pieces to the puzzle. Our food supply is part of the problem, so are our food choices. Lifestyle is another one. We're living at such a fast, stressful pace and we don't have much time to spend in the kitchen and end up grabbing whatever we can. Our relationship with food is also a big issue. It's really for the purpose of nourishing and fueling our bodies but it has become much more to most of us – our friend, our lover, our comforter, even our God.

Are you ready to go on a journey? Is gaining a healthy, vibrant body important enough to you to set aside some time for learning what is necessary to make it happen? I'm not going to hand you a food plan and tell you to stick with it and then you'll lose X pounds a week. You can find countless books and programs that will tell you that despite the fact that they frequently contradict one another. We're going to walk hand in hand through this discovery process and create a plan just for you.

If your mind is made up, come with me.

What do you do when you know you're going on a trip? Let's assume you're going from Denver to Chicago by car. Would you plan your itinerary and look at a roadmap and figure out the best way to get there? What will you do if you encounter bad weather? How much money will you need? How will you handle detours? Did you allow enough time? What will you do if someone tries to talk you into going somewhere else? Would you find a city that's halfway there and make a motel reservation? Would you pick out places to stop along the way for meals or taking a break? Would you prepare the car, filling it up with gas, checking the oil and fan belts, washing it maybe? Would you decide what clothes to take based on the activities you would be involved in, making sure they were clean and then packing them neatly? Would you have done research on the Internet or looked at brochures to see what's there? Would you pack snacks for the trip and take a book to read in the motel or some CD's to listen to?

Let's assume that you are so excited about going to Chicago that you just run out to your car, jump in and start driving. You head east because you know that Chicago is in that general direction. So you're bebopping along and you get a ways down the road and realize that you're about out of gas. You find a gas station and start to fill up and realize that you don't have enough cash. So you have to use your credit card which you had vowed not to use anymore. Oh well, what choice do you have? You really want to go to Chicago. You also realize you're hungry and there's nothing in the gas station store except chips and cookies. There aren't any restaurants around so once again you eat something unhealthy, shrugging your shoulders. Who can blame you? You really want to get to Chicago and you didn't have time to prepare snacks. Getting on the road was the most important thing, wasn't it? So you're on the road again, stuffing chips and cookies and drinking soda pop and you see this huge billboard advertising Florida. There's the ocean with palm trees and the sun shining. Wow, that looks good! Maybe Chicago is not such a great choice after all. It can be cold and windy there and not too sunny. Florida looks so enticing. What would a little detour hurt? You can always go to Chicago later. So you take the road leading to Florida and spend a few days on the beach. But then a hurricane comes and just about wipes you out. You flee for your life and head for Chicago again. You're now sunburned and hung over from all the Pina Coladas you drank by the pool plus you're bloated and feeling sluggish from all the rich food that the hotel had to offer. Chicago is suddenly looking good again. You had forgotten that they have a beautiful lake, lots of museums and other interesting attractions plus you have some good friends there that you've really been wanting to see again. It's been a long time since you were together.

So now you're headed north toward Chicago and feeling better about yourself. You're not sure you're on the right highway but you figure you'll see a sign sooner or later that will indicate what's up ahead. Your clothes are getting grungy because they're the only ones you brought but you shrug again and decide to buy some more when you get there. After all, they have great shopping there! Yes, you'll have to use your credit card again which is already straining from the overload but after all, you don't really have a choice, do you? A little ways down the road you see a billboard for Texas. There's the Alamo, cowboys, great Mexican food, and friendly people. You know, that might be better than Chicago. At least for a few days...

Are you getting it? Do you see how important it is to know exactly where you're going, why you want to go there, how to get there, what the journey might be like and what preparations to make for the journey? This is absolutely key!

It is highly unlikely that you will get to Chicago if you're just joyriding all over the U.S.

This assignment will be ongoing because you don't know all the answers yet. The first thing to decide is where you are going. What is your Chicago? Visualize what you want your life to look like – not just your weight or health but everything else including your work, relationships, financial situation, attitude, spiritual life, etc. What pictures do you see in your head when you think about it? Why do you want these things? What's the attraction? Why do you want to go there?

Next is what will get you there. We will be discussing some of those things in this book but some of them will be for you to decide. The vehicle in which you travel is very important so getting healthy and fit is a big key to achieving many of your other goals.

What preparations do you need to make for this trip? Are you willing to give them top priority and schedule them into your day – every day? If your desire to get to Chicago isn't strong enough you will always be taking detours to some other destination. If Florida and Texas aren't on the way to Chicago from Denver then why would you go there?

A great way to keep your vision before you is to make a Dream Board. Get a piece of poster board in whatever size you desire and start cutting out pictures and words from magazines that are indicative of your goals. Once you've got enough of them, paste them onto the board in a collage and hang it on the wall in a place you'll see it every day. Make sure that it covers all aspects of your life. This will take awhile to complete but at least get started on it. Visualization, as well as writing, can be very powerful tools. The mind loves imagery and symbolism and latches on to it.

Get some preliminary writing done on your destination before going to the next chapter. It will help you make other decisions. After all, if I was going to Chicago in the winter I wouldn't take a bikini unless I was going to stay in a hotel with an indoor pool and hot tub.

What are your goals? Start making a list of everything you want to achieve and when. Health is about your whole life not just your weight. After you've made your list I want you to visualize what this would look like. Our imaginations are a powerful tool. See yourself healthy, vibrant, slender, fit, prosperous, living out your dream. If you can't see it in your mind then it's not likely to manifest. Write a scenario of how your ideal life would look when you obtain these goals but write it in the present tense as if it had already happened. Don't let the mean nag in your head tell you that you can't do it or any other nonsense. See the picture in your mind and then start writing. As you write it will grow and you will get more information about it and get more excited. You can rewrite it as many times as you want. The first time I wrote about my ideal life in Texas (while I was still in Colorado) it didn't ring true. I realized that I was writing it according to what I thought someone else wanted me to do and so I rewrote it with the truth that was in me. It felt right and I didn't need to make any more revisions. Since then I've written some new things that spawned from that first scenario. It is absolutely essential that you set aside all the messages coming at you from your head and other people. When you've reached your truth you'll feel it in your heart.

Buy a special journal to write in if it helps. I use a spiral notebook but I write with a beautiful red Waterman fountain pen that I bought in Vienna. Although I'm writing this book on my laptop all my journaling is by hand. It just seems to work better that way and I can take it anywhere.

Let's get going!

Chapter 4
Blueprint for Change

So how do we change? I don't know about you but I have tried to change various things countless times and been defeated. It's very frustrating when you get yourself all psyched up and eager to begin a new diet or exercise program and then end up blowing it before the end of the day. What happened?

It all starts with words – the words coming into our ears and the words coming out of our mouths. Words are seeds and will sprout and grow according to their kind. If you plant watermelon seeds you get watermelon. If you plant marigold seeds you get marigolds. If you plant negative words you get negative thinking. If you plant positive words you get positive thinking. What have you been planting?

Words in turn influence your thinking. The thoughts whirling in your brain are there because you or someone else planted them. How does your garden grow? Have you been allowing weeds to take it over? Have you been planting good seed, watering and fertilizing it? Or do you let just any old thing take root in you and grow? Your body, spirit, and mind need a caretaker just like a garden does. If you wouldn't allow anyone to touch your body inappropriately why would you allow someone to touch your mind and spirit inappropriately? Worse yet, why would you do it to yourself?

Your thinking affects your emotions. When someone compliments and praises you, how do you feel? Doesn't it instantly boost your mood and self-esteem? You feel lighter and happier and you're able to be more productive or be more loving toward yourself and others. What happens when someone insults or disparages you? You may feel anger toward them and hurt but don't you also start doubting and feeling bad about yourself? Your mood plummets and you drag your feet and look at the ground. You couldn't care less about anyone else because you've stopped loving yourself. You lose all desire to do anything productive or positive. You just want to go curl up in a dark corner. Emotions get you in motion either forward or backward.

You have to get rid of your "stinking thinking" before you can feel better. You are responsible for changing how you think and feel. You are the one who has the choice of what you say, hear and see. Put a guard on your eye gate, ear gate, and mouth gate. If you don't like what you're feeling, change what you're thinking and saying. Don't go looking for somebody else (or some food) to make you feel better. It's just temporary and can make you feel worse afterwards. Don't give away your power. You are the CEO of yourself. Don't let some flunky boss you around. Take a tip from Donald Trump and say "You're fired, flunky. I'm running the show now."

You can see how your feelings can influence your actions. When you first get excited about a new diet or exercise program you're all energized and ready to do it. That may sustain you for awhile but if your words and feeling go sour then your positive actions stop also. If you start telling yourself that it's too hard or too much trouble or you don't have enough time or whatever then your actions follow suit. Next thing you know you're sitting on the sofa eating bon-bons and watching the food channel on TV. Everything came to a screeching halt and all you did was change what you were saying to yourself and made a decision based on those words. A decision comes before an action. It doesn't just happen. You decided, no one else.

When you've done the same thing for a long enough period of time then it becomes a habit – either good or bad. It took a lot of repetition for it to become automatic and it didn't happen overnight. You won't change it overnight. Creating a good habit requires a lot of repetition also and you can't give up just because it didn't work the first time. The worst thing you can do is start telling yourself what an idiot you are or how hopeless you are, blah, blah, blah. Those words will start your feet moving down the wrong road again. If you took an off ramp that leads away from your chosen destination then find the next turnaround and get headed back in the right direction. I don't care how many times you have to turn around, just do it. If you decided you wanted to go to Chicago then Florida is not an option. List all the reasons you want to go there and post the list in many visible places where you'll see it frequently.

Are you the kind of person who keeps commitments? Do you keep them to yourself also? Arriving at your destination is about more than reaching your goal weight or becoming muscular and fit. You are developing your character as you go. Making decisions that are for your highest good and putting them into action will make you become the kind of person who keeps commitments, gets things done, influences and leads others, etc. People will want to be around you and seek you out. You'll feel good about yourself and others will feel good about themselves just being around you because you always speak positive and seek to impart it to others.

It's all about the journey and who you become while you're on it. Once you reach your destination it won't be long before you'll be picking another destination that's even farther down the road. The vehicle you drive and the toolkit you carry are very important. Preparation is essential. We don't want to be running out of gas just a few miles down the road or eating stale crackers at a roadside stand. Before we delve into health education we'll take a look at the items that need to go into our toolkit.

Chapter 5
Toolkit

Food Diary – you will need to write down everything you eat and how you felt.

Journal – this is very important. You will be writing down your goals, visions, longings, difficulties, thoughts, emotions, etc.

Dream board – this is a visual reminder of where you want to go and what you want your life to be like.

Goals – a written list of where you're going, your destination.

Spiritual practice – you will definitely need to spend time with God every day. You can't do this under your own power. You've already tried that, remember?

How this looks and what it consists of depends upon your beliefs, your level of commitment and the amount of time you have available.

Food plan – we're going to be putting this together as we go through the chapters. It will be unique to you.

Exercise schedule and equipment – we'll be talking about this more. Start with what you can and keep adding to it.

Alternate plans – write out a plan for how you will handle different situations such as eating out, cravings, being too tired to cook, parties, etc. We'll be talking about that some more and it can change as you grow in knowledge and experience.

Support team – enlist friends or family who will be supportive of you. Someone who will let you share from your heart and not encourage you to drown your sorrows in food. Choose someone who is uplifting and will cheer you on.

Books, CDs, DVDs – have plenty of positive educational and inspirational literature on hand that you can read or listen to daily to keep you encouraged.

Affirmations – keep a list of positive statements about yourself (I like to base mine on Bible verses). Speak them out loud to yourself every day to build up your belief level and to remind yourself of the truth.

Chapter 6
Toxemia and Nutritional Deficiency

The bottom line where health is concerned is what goes in and what comes out. You need a clean body in which to put optimum nutrition otherwise the nutrients won't be absorbed. Toxicity creates many other problems also.

Toxemia is a term used to describe poisons that are stored in the body. Where do we get these toxins? They come from the air, household chemicals, personal care products, cosmetics, and our food. Yes, our food is poisoned. Our meat and dairy contain antibiotics and hormones. Produce is sprayed with insecticides. Toxins get stored in our fat cells in our body's attempt to protect us. Our bodies are also holding on to excess water in an effort to dilute the poisons. It's no wonder we're bloated and can't shed the extra pounds.

As if that wasn't bad enough, most people are malnourished. Our soils are so depleted of minerals that produce only has a fraction of the nutrients in it that it had in the early 1900s. Or it could be due to a digestive problem which prevents nutrients from being absorbed efficiently. Or microorganisms like Candida Albicans (yeast) that grab the nutrients before they reach the bloodstream so your body is still screaming for food even though your stomach is full. Candida love sugar and starch and they never get enough. And the more you feed them the more they'll punish you by causing all sorts of health problems. What ingratitude!! Also, when you eat a high fat diet it is harder for the glucose to get into the cells so all that sugar keeps circulating in your bloodstream – more for the Candida to snack on!

Allergies are another cause of overeating. A strong daily craving for a particular food could be an indication that you're allergic to it. And the more you eat the more you crave it. After many years, I finally made the connection between sugar and refined starches and my headaches, mood swings and fatigue. It takes at least three days to clear your body of a food, sometimes a little longer. When I'm free from sugar, flour and wheat my appetite drops drastically. That doesn't mean that I don't think about those foods but at least my cells aren't screaming for them. I become interested in healthier foods and I get full quicker. Unfortunately, sugar, flour and wheat are so prevalent in our foods that I have to be really careful or I'll accidentally eat something that will trigger a headache and cravings. So I've had to learn to read labels and when I eat out I quiz the servers about ingredients. They usually don't know the answer and have to go ask the chef. There is frequently sugar in the salad dressing and MSG and possibly flour or sugar in the seasonings they put on meat. Soups, sauces and gravies are thickened with flour. You have to be vigilant!

There are also preservatives and additives in our foods that are synthetic chemicals. Some of them are to keep the food from spoiling so it will have a long shelf life. Who wants old food? The additives are there to add flavor but some of them are excitotoxins such as MSG. They excite the cells to death and make you want more at the same time. If it's real food why would we need to add flavor and why would we want more than our bodies need? Obviously, we wouldn't but the manufacturers would. They want us to eat the whole bag of chips, not just one. Packaged and restaurant foods are also over salted so of course your body has to hold on to extra water to dilute it.

So we need to start cleansing our bodies of the toxins while we work on transitioning to better food choices. Because your body will start detoxing as soon as you change your food for the better we'll wait on other detoxification methods until later. The toxins will take their revenge on you for giving them their walking papers. You may have some discomfort while they're departing. Headaches, fatigue, achy body, nausea, and excess mucous could be some of the symptoms you might feel. Just remember, you're not getting sick, you're getting better because you're cleaning out your body. After about three days you'll start feeling better. You may have additional healing responses in the future as your body continues to cleanse itself of years of toxins. Just remind yourself that it's temporary.

Drinking lots of water will speed the process. You should be drinking half your weight in ounces of water a day. Example – if you weight 150 lbs., drink 75 oz. of water. If you're not drinking much now start slowly and build up. It is also imperative that your bowels move regularly. We really should be eliminating after every meal but because of our refined foods and not enough fiber and water we are lucky if we go once a day. Don't take fiber supplements until you get things moving more because they could stop you up more. You can take magnesium which hydrates the bowel or some herbal laxatives. Eating more high water and fiber content foods like fruits and vegetables is going to help also. We don't want those toxins hanging around in a clogged up bowel causing more trouble. They could be reabsorbed into the body. Colon cleanses are very beneficial. You may email me for recommendations.

Now it's time to start making our changes. The first thing that needs to go is refined sugar. It has no nutritional value at all and contributes to obesity, cancer, diabetes, etc. and robs your body of other nutrients. One teaspoon of sugar can suppress your immune system for up to eight hours. And forget artificial sweeteners – they're definitely poison. You might be okay with raw honey, maple syrup or some other food-based sweeteners but for now it's better to get rid of it entirely. You can use stevia which is plant-based. You can find it in health food stores, just follow the directions on the package. When you want something sweet, have fruit. Fresh fruit, not cooked or canned. Raw foods contain living enzymes that help us digest the food. Heat over 115°F kills the enzymes.

Add a salad to your meals every day. Dark, leafy greens as a base with numerous choices of raw vegetables on top – broccoli, cauliflower, tomatoes, radishes, carrots, celery, zucchini, peppers (red, yellow or gold, not green), onions, etc. I actually like most vegetables raw better than cooked. I also sometimes add beans, pumpkin seeds, sunflower seeds, or walnuts if I'm making a meal of it or even boiled eggs, cheese or meat if I'm not eating vegan. (A vegan doesn't eat any meat products at all.) A nice simple dressing in small amounts is all you need. It's really easy to make your own and it tastes so much better. Have you ever read the label on those bottled ones? Yuck!

If adding raw fruit and salad to your diet gives you digestion difficulties it may take a while for your body to adjust. You may need to take some food enzymes and probiotics (the good bacteria) to help with that. The probiotics are necessary and will be covered in the next chapter.

It will also be helpful if you can start buying organic food to avoid adding more chemicals to your body. If you can't get organic produce then wash it very well with a cleanser for that purpose. You can find food washes in the grocery store, usually in the produce section.

When you're grocery shopping learn to be a detective. You must read labels. If you don't recognize the name you probably shouldn't be eating it. Better yet, don't buy anything that's packaged or processed. Fresh produce and whole grains haven't been processed. Refined grains have had most of the nutrients refined right out of them. When you buy nuts and seeds make sure they are raw and not roasted.

As you change your diet for the better your body will finally have what it needs to build new healthy cells and it can let go of the old diseased ones and all the toxins it's been holding on to. As they head out of your body through your elimination channels – kidneys, bowels, lungs, skin – they might possibly punish you on the way out. That's why it's important to get them out quickly by having your bowels moving regularly (optimally, after every meal) and your kidneys working freely. The water and high fiber food will help flush them out. There are colon cleanses and other types of detoxification programs but you don't want to overload yourself. My favorite detoxification protocol is the IonCleanse® footbath which gently pulls toxins from your body using charged particles called ions. The ions enter through the pores of your feet, go into your whole body, latch onto oppositely charged particles, and pull them back out into the water.

What you breathe and put on your skin is just as important as what you put into your body. It all gets into your tissues. Don't use artificial air fresheners, perfumes and chemical-based cleansers in your home. I realize you can't do anything about the outside air or all the out-gassing that your home and furniture are doing. But you don't have to add to it! Buy the detergents and household cleaners that are chemical free. You may email me for recommendations.

I grew up in a farming community and one Sunday afternoon I was exposed to airborne pesticides twice. They were crop dusting over our house and then we went to my sister's house and they were at it there too. By the next day my sinuses were gushing mucus in an attempt to rid my body of the poison. I didn't know anything about natural remedies back then. I suffered through it all week and ended up with a bad sinus infection and went to the doctor and got antibiotics which, of course, gave me a yeast infection. I was a mess. And as a result of growing up surrounded by farm chemicals I have always had allergies to chemicals and strong chemical odors. If I encounter a strong paint smell I will not stay in that room because I'll end up with a headache or gushing sinuses. So I'm really careful what I breathe now.

Shampoos, body lotions, skin care products, cosmetics, toothpaste, etc. are full of carcinogens and chemicals. If you can't eat it you don't want it on your skin because it will still get into all your cells. You can easily find chemical free personal care products in health food stores and some grocery stores or you can email me for some excellent product recommendations.

Drink filtered water. We need to keep our bodies hydrated but we don't need chlorine and fluoride. There are better ways of preventing dental cavities – like eating a healthy, whole food diet.

In addition, keep a food diary every day. Write down what you've eaten and if you have time, how you felt physically, mentally and spiritually. Even if it's just a few words it will be helpful to you in the future for determining habits and patterns that have an effect on you. This was how I discovered the foods that I'm allergic to and the ways they impacted me. Remember, you're removing refined sugar and eating raw fruit instead, adding salads every day and drinking half your weight in ounces of water.

Chapter 7
Bacteria – The Good, The Bad, and The Ugly

It has been said by many in the natural healing world that "Death begins in the colon". Societies that practiced eating fermented foods and special bacterial cultures called kefirs have been found to live long lives. There is definitely a link between human longevity and maintaining a healthy balance of bacteria in the body.

The bacteria in our digestive tracts all serve a purpose but when the "bad" bacteria are out of balance with the "good" bacteria then trouble starts. The ideal ratio of friendly bacteria to pathogenic bacteria is 85% probiotic bacteria to 15% pathogenic bacteria. But the opposite is what most people have. When you suffer from low quantities of good bacteria your immune system is severely compromised. This leaves you predisposed to fatigue, joint inflammation, viral attack, parasites, allergies and all manner of digestive disorders and life-threatening diseases.

The common warning signs of a bacterial imbalance include:

- Difficulty losing weight, sugar/starch cravings
- Fatigue, poor concentration and memory
- Constipation or diarrhea
- Indigestion, acid reflux, heartburn and other digestive disorders
- Sleeping poorly, night sweats
- Painful joint inflammation and stiffness
- Bad breath, gum disease, thrush
- Frequent colds, flu or infections
- Chronic yeast problems, Candida overgrowth
- Acne, eczema, skin and foot fungus
- Extreme menstrual or menopausal symptoms
- Allergies and food sensitivities

We are exposed to billions of tons of pollutants in our everyday lives. As our toxin levels rise and go unchecked, our immune system and other critical processes in our body become dangerously compromised and begin to fail.

Bacteria are at the base of all life on this planet and they produce enzymes. These enzymes then identify, digest and deliver nutrients where they need to go. Your cells need enzymes to function correctly. Enzymes are responsible for every metabolic process in your body and if there is a deficit of friendly (probiotic) bacteria in the human gut, then there is a deficit of enzymes. Without these vital enzymes, nutrients do not get used. This lack of uptake of nutrients is behind the causes of most of the disorders of the human body. You can consume the best nutrients in the world but if you cannot digest and assimilate them they aren't being used by your body.

Things that kill bacteria in the body:

- Antibiotics
- Birth control pills
- Steroidal/hormonal drugs
- Fluoride, Chlorine
- Coffee, tea, carbonated drinks
- Manmade vitamins
- Synthetic ascorbic acid
- Radiation
- Stress
- Preservatives, additives
- Pesticides, fertilizers

It's very important to choose a probiotic supplement that contains a wide spectrum of bacteria as well as a delivery mechanism that enables them to survive until they get to your intestines. Taking probiotics regularly will keep the population of bad bacteria under control. Probiotics will help prevent the invasion of harmful bacteria, yeasts, molds, viruses and parasites. With a reduced number of unfriendly bacteria there will be fewer toxic substances (excreted by them) that leave the colon and get absorbed into the bloodstream. You may email me for recommendations of the best ones to use.

Chapter 8
Enzymes – The Life of Foods

Cooked foods are dead foods. If you don't believe me try putting both a raw potato and a cooked potato in the ground and see which one sprouts. Raw and living foods contain enzymes which are substances which make life possible. They are needed for every chemical reaction that occurs in our bodies. Without enzymes, no activity at all would take place. Vitamins, minerals nor hormones can do any work without enzymes.

Our bodies are made up of living cells and they need living food to nourish them. Live foods contain life force. A diet of at least 75% raw vegetarian foods including fruit, vegetables, nuts, seeds and sprouted grains has been credited with enabling your body to heal itself of acne, allergies, arthritis, asthma, diabetes, depression, fibromyalgia, gallstones, hair loss, hearing loss, high blood pressure, high cholesterol, obesity, and much more. The extra amounts of vitamins, minerals, enzymes and fiber along with reduced calorie consumption and more balanced blood sugar, speed raw foodists toward lean good health. Raw vegetables, for example, have been found to contain 77% more B6, 86.5% more Vitamin E, and up to 40% more zinc than cooked vegetables.

Enzymes are important because they assist in the digestion and absorption of food. When you eat dead food your body will not get maximum utilization of the food. The three primary digestive enzymes are protease, lipase and amylase which digest, respectively, protein, fat, and carbohydrates. Carbohydrates include fruits, vegetables, grains and sugars.

There aren't any across the board rules for everyone. We're all different in our bodies and level of health and many are not ready mentally and emotionally to embrace such a huge change in their diet and lifestyle. It can take months or years to gradually make the transition to healthier foods while learning more about it. It's best for people to start at the level they can manage and begin building from there, adding the live foods and subtracting the dead ones.

If you are ill you may need to be on a 100% raw food diet for awhile. If you are well you can eat 75% raw foods (fruits, vegetables, dark, leafy greens) and a maximum of 25% cooked foods like steamed vegetables and whole grains. Some people even include a little meat and dairy in the cooked portion. You really can get all the protein you need from this diet and you can get the high quality fat from small amounts of avocados and soaked nuts and seeds.

If all this is starting to seem overwhelming I have good news. You don't have to learn it all at once. After all, you didn't learn how to "cook" all at once. You probably started out boiling water. Just eating more fruit and salads is a great place to start. Just don't load up with unhealthy, fatty dressings. One of my favorite ways to get more raw food is a green smoothie. I know it sounds strange but it's really yummy. You don't have to be real exact with your measurements either. One I make frequently in my blender starts with 2 cups of water, a banana, two handfuls of organic baby spinach and some frozen blueberries to make it thick and cold. I also love the combination of mangoes and strawberries or papayas and pineapple I sometimes add a packet of stevia for sweetener or you could add raw honey or agave nectar. Depending on what fruit is in season and available I'll change it around. You can always find organic frozen fruit. I like to buy the already washed organic baby spinach and lettuces because they're so much easier. If you decide to use the stronger greens such as kale, collards, chard, etc. add a lemon or lime to get rid of the bitterness.

Don't let your salads be the same old boring lettuce and tomatoes. Use the dark, leafy greens, not iceberg. Instead of automatically cooking your vegetables, put them in your salad instead. Top it with a few walnuts – they contain those great

Omega 3 fats. Use a light vinaigrette dressing or just squeeze lemon on your salad. Use a variety of colors to make it more attractive and to get a wider array of nutrients. There's a whole lot more to learn and have fun with but that's a good start.

Vibrant health is not just for a few lucky people. It can be you too. Choose life!

When and if you eat cooked food it is very important to take food enzyme supplements. Get one that includes the enzymes mentioned above along with HCl (hydrochloric acid). Many people are deficient in HCl without realizing it and they're popping antacids to calm down the heartburn and indigestion when the problem is really the opposite – they need more HCl, not less.

Chapter 9
Get Off the Roller Coaster

When you eat sugar and refined starches it causes your blood sugar to go on a roller coaster ride. The pancreas gets worn out trying to keep up with the insulin required to escort the glucose into your cells. Also, if you eat a high fat diet it will inhibit that process also. It is not my purpose here to explain how your body works. You can read a biology textbook for that. I just want to point out that eating non-food items (I don't consider refined foods to be real food) will cause your body to become unbalanced and will not give you the nutrients required for optimum health and life.

Blood sugar disorders have become epidemic (diabetes, hypoglycemia) in this country, even among children. This is due in part to our excess consumption of refined sweets, flour products and fatty foods. We also don't consume enough fiber to slow down the rush of these sugars into our bloodstream.

Whole foods contain both a wide spectrum of nutrients and the fiber needed to slow down the absorption process. Refined sugars and starches also lead to the bacterial imbalance mentioned in the previous chapter. Refined foods get bogged down in your colon because of lack of fiber and water, leading to fermentation and constipation. Craving sugars and starches can be a result of both blood sugar imbalances and Candida overgrowth.

Beware of other names for sugar like high fructose corn syrup, sucrose, fructose. Even honey and maple syrup are still basically sugar. If you can't eat any of those items without a reaction or bingeing then just avoid them. All it takes is one little bite to send you down the road to overeating. The sugar alcohols (like mannitol, sorbitol, xylitol) that have become so popular will give you gas and diarrhea. Who wants that?

So just forget the refined stuff. Many of the vitamins contained in whole grains have been milled out. Eat real food: whole grains such as oats, buckwheat, quinoa, barley, amaranth, kamut, teff, etc. If you have to have bread eat sprouted grain bread. You can find it in the freezer section of most grocery stores. They even make sprouted grain tortillas! A health food store will usually have the largest selection. But you'll want to go easy on the grains. After all, that's how they fatten up livestock before slaughter. Instead of pasta eat small amounts of starchy vegetables such as sweet potatoes, butternut squash, or acorn squash. Just don't load on the butter. If you just have to have spaghetti then pour your sauce over grated raw vegetables such as zucchini or cooked spaghetti squash. You can even make raw spaghetti and lasagna! Take a look at the suggested recipe books in Appendix B.

There is absolutely no food value in refined sugar products. Face it – you're just indulging yourself, you're not nourishing yourself. If that's what you choose to do then go ahead but don't lie to yourself. Food spells comfort to a lot of people and it can become their God. Have you been worshipping in the candy or bakery aisles of the supermarket? Just eat fruit!

In addition to removing flour products from your diet and adding whole grain and/or sprouted grain products, add more vegetables. You should be eating at least one small salad a day by now. Add another one. You can have it for breakfast if you want but I'd suggest lunch and dinner. Eat it first. Unless it's really huge have some more vegetables on the side with your meat or whatever you're having. Your vegetables should occupy one half of your plate, your meat or protein one fourth and your starchy vegetable or whole grain one fourth (if you just absolutely have to have a starch). A salad should precede the meal or be that one half of your plate. You'll be too full for dessert!

Refined foods have been stripped of many of their nutrients and due to mineral depletion of our soils even the best of food isn't always enough. Most people will need nutritional supplementation. I have seen supplements make a huge difference in people's health. It will be different for each individual, though. Different bodies have different nutritional needs. See Appendix A for more information. You may email me with questions about the products.

Chapter 10
Is It Hot In Here or Is It Just Me?

Estrogen dominance has become a huge problem in the U.S. How did this happen? Xenoestrogens (xeno means new or foreign) are everywhere, most manmade as by-products of industrial or food production. They are in your plastic cup, computer chips, PVC piping, soap, clothes, pharmaceuticals, detergents and household cleaners, pesticides, fertilizers, meat, dairy, unfiltered water, cosmetics, skin and personal care products and so on. We are eating, drinking, breathing and slathering on our skin harmful substances. So not only are they making us fat they're also unbalancing our hormones and permeating our cells, leading to the breakdown of our immune systems. Research is finding that the animal kingdom is being affected as well as humans. How are xenoestrogens affecting humans?

- In the past 100 years the average age of menarche (the first menstrual flow) dropped from age 16 to 12.
- About 30% of women with endometriosis are infertile.
- Breast cancer strikes 1 in 8 women, up from 1 in 30 just a generation ago.
- Male sperm counts continue to drop in the U.S. population.
- Increasing numbers of young boys are reporting development of female secondary sex characteristics, with delayed development of male characteristics.
- 600,000–1,000,000 women have hysterectomies every year. Of these surgeries, 90% are unnecessary.

For women, using progesterone cream (made from plants) can bring your hormones back into balance. There are also herbs such as black cohosh, dong quai, red clover, and red raspberry that have been found to be helpful. Both the cream and the herbs can be found in supermarkets as well as drugstores and health food stores and include instructions for their use. Or you can just change your food. I found that removing sugar, flour and chemicals from my diet solved the problem for me.

Eating a toxic, refined diet will definitely affect your hormones also. I can speak from personal experience. When I eat sugar, flour, wheat or non-organic foods I will not only get a headache but I will have hot flashes and insomnia. It will be different for everyone but it's certainly something to notice about yourself. If you've been diligently writing in your journals you may have started to notice some patterns. If you haven't it may just take a while. You'll learn to be a detective.

Phytoestrogens are found primarily in plants. When you eat plants like spinach, lettuces, beans and legumes, fruits, soy products and flaxseed you get ample amounts of phytoestrogens. They can fill the estrogen receptor, satisfying the body's need for estrogen stimulation, while actually blocking a stronger estrogen (xenoestrogens) that may try to enter the receptor with a more harmful message. Fiber is also a great estrogen fighter. Estrogen is excreted in the stool and if it remains in the body too long it will be reabsorbed.

My favorite food remedy for hormonal issues is flaxseed. Not the oil but the whole seeds, bought fresh and kept refrigerated because they go rancid very easily. You need to grind it fresh yourself each time because the meal will go bad even faster than the seeds. All you need is an electric coffee grinder. Don't use it for anything else! Start with a teaspoon a day and work your way up to the amount that feels right to your body (2–3 Tbsp.). Flaxseeds contain phytoestrogens which help normalize your hormones and fight the effects of the chemical-based estrogens that are everywhere. This is effective for both men and women. They will also give you both much-needed fiber and some good fats such as Omega 3.

Chapter 11
Not All Fats Are the Bad Guys

Fats are not all bad. Your body needs fats to deliver vitamins, regulate cholesterol metabolism, cushion your vital organs and give you healthy skin and energy. They also play an important part in protecting us from heart disease.

Yes, there are unhealthy fats and they should be reduced in your diet. The easiest way to figure out if it's okay to eat it is to avoid cooked fat like fried foods and processed foods that contain hydrogenated fats. The good fats found in fish, extra virgin olive oil, avocadoes, nuts and seeds can improve blood cholesterol levels, lower your risk for heart disease, help suppress hunger and make you stronger at the cellular level. Most people get enough of the Omega 6 fats and not enough of the Omega 3s. Omega 3 essential fatty acids are found in fish oil, flaxseed, and walnuts mostly. Flaxseeds are my favorite source because they also help with hormones and fiber. I do not like fish oil supplements because it's too easy for them to go rancid. It's better to just eat more fish if you're not a vegetarian. Eat wild caught fish, not farm raised because they have fewer toxins. There is no pure food left in the world so don't get too hung up on perfection. Just try to make the best choice.

Omega-3 (DHA and EPA) fatty acids have been shown to lower the risk of heart disease and potentially reduce prostate cancer incidence. Omega-3 fatty acids actually help strengthen the membranes around your billions of body cells, making you stronger at the cellular level. Additionally, DHA and EPA help reduce the amount of cholesterol the liver makes and they thin the blood, making clots less likely to form in arterial plaque.

Refined fat and oil products are nutritionally equivalent to refined white sugars and white flour in carbohydrate nutrition – empty calories. They cannot be properly digested and metabolized, they rob our body of its stores of minerals and vitamins, and they lead to deficiency of essential nutrients and fatty degeneration.

Trans-fatty acids are produced by high temperatures and hydrogenation that turn refined oils into margarines, shortenings, shortening oils, and partially hydrogenated vegetable oils. Trans-fatty acids are not good for your body. They have been associated with many diseases such as atherosclerosis and cancer.

Virgin or extra-virgin olive oils are good but are low in essential fatty acids so you will also need to add flaxseed or fish oil to your diet to obtain those. Hemp oil has a better ratio of Omega 6s to Omega 3s than flax. I prefer to use the freshly ground flaxseed as opposed to the oil because it will be fresher.

Chapter 12
To Eat or Not to Eat Meat??

For decades we have been told by the meat, dairy and egg industries that we need their products to get enough protein and calcium. I'm not saying you have to become a vegetarian if you choose not to but you don't need the huge quantities that they claim. There is plenty of protein and calcium in plants along with many vitamins and minerals that you don't find in meat and dairy. A lot of vegetarians aren't even eating vegetables and fruit all that much. They're eating non-meat items like pasta, bread and desserts and those are the worst things you can eat. Both the meat eaters and the vegetarians tend to eat too many refined grain and sugar products and not enough vegetables and fruits.

The biggest problem with meat and dairy are the hormones given to cows to increase milk production and the antibiotics given to animals to fight the diseases they develop because of the horrible conditions they're raised under. Most of them are kept in cages where they become extremely toxic from overcrowding and inactivity. If you're going to eat meat and dairy, eat organic and try to find some that is free range. Yes, it's more expensive but it's better than poisoning your body.

The second problem is getting an excess of protein. Meat and dairy can be acid-forming in the body for a lot of people and your body will take calcium from your bones to keep your blood pH stable. Osteoporosis isn't caused from lack of milk or Tums because those aren't viable sources of calcium. Cow's milk is meant for calves – do you want to get that big and have hooves? Goat's milk is closer to the composition of human milk. And milk is meant for babies, not adults. Dairy products are high in fat also so moderation is advised.

Foods like dark leafy greens, almonds, sesame seeds and kelp are high in calcium and the body can utilize them better.

Many people can also get plenty of protein from a vegan diet of fruits, vegetables, nuts, seeds, and sprouts. Some people may need some meat or fish in their diet and some may not. It's an individual thing and you will have to experiment on yourself to find out.

Your next transition is to eat less meat and dairy and eat more fish, nuts, and seeds. The fish should be wild and not farm raised. It's hard to find unpolluted fish regardless of its origin. Don't overdo the nuts and seeds because they are high in calories. They will be more digestible if you soak them in pure water overnight. Then rinse and drain. They will need to be kept in the refrigerator. Or you can re-dry them using a dehydrator and keeping the temperature under 115°F. Nuts and seeds contain phytates that inhibit sprouting under normal conditions. Those phytates also make them harder to digest. Once you've soaked or even sprouted them they are easier to digest and easier on your teeth too!

If you are lactose intolerant and want substitutes for dairy there are many recipes for using nuts and seeds to make milks, cheeses, yogurts, etc. They won't taste just like dairy but are an acceptable substitute. Nuts and seeds are high in fat, though, so moderation is advised if you need to lose weight. See Appendix B for a list of some of my favorite recipe books, both cooked and raw.

Chapter 13
What's Eating Me?

Keep journaling about your issues surrounding making all these changes. Ask God for insight concerning these issues. You need to get to the root of your resistance. The battle is won or lost in our minds. What we think about consistently is the direction our emotions and beliefs will go. We don't have to think about whatever pops into our head. We can kick it out and substitute something positive. What is the underlying cause or thread running through our rebellion and unwillingness to give up our crutches? What gaping hole are we trying to fill? Not enough love from our family and friends, lack of fulfilling work, anxiety over money, getting older, feeling like a failure, the list goes on.

Victory comes first on the inside before it shows on the outside. You have to be careful what you allow in your mind just like you want to only put healthy food in your body. You wouldn't drink gasoline, would you? There are a lot of things we allow into our mind that ignite a fire that can be very difficult to put out. When you're thinking about a sweet treat does the thought just go away by itself or does it consume you completely until you run to the kitchen or store to satisfy the urge? When you have a negative thought about yourself do you kick it out right away or dwell on it until you're wallowing in self-hatred or self-pity? Instead, substitute some thoughts that light a good fire. Remind yourself where you're going and picture again and again what it's going to look and feel like when you get there. The pull toward your goal needs to be stronger than the pull toward the doughnut. Pray for strength and guidance. You may need to utilize a coach or counselor to help you root out the deeper issues that are keeping you from moving forward. I work with people one-on-one to coach and support them through their journey.

God's word is full of positive words about His love for us and how He wants to bless us and help us grow. Pick some verses that address your situation and write them on index cards or sticky notes. Put them everywhere so you will see them and eventually you'll have them memorized so they'll pop into your mind at the appropriate time. Listening to scripture set to music has been very helpful to me in learning it. When you're in your car don't listen to the junk on the radio. Listen to motivational or educational tapes that will build you up. Don't be a prisoner of your mind. You can control what goes into it.

Whatever you're thinking about all the time will come out in your words and actions. Your actions get you to your goal. Spend some time writing about your actions and where you will end up if you keep doing the same thing you've always done. Then write about which actions you need to do to get you to your desired goal. Make sure you implement them into your daily life.

Chapter 14
Why Exercise?

Our bodies were meant to move, not sit on our rear ends in front of a TV or computer all day. We not only need exercise every day but we need a variety so we don't get bored. It doesn't take long for our bodies to start declining in strength, energy and flexibility when we don't exercise.

Aerobic exercise will help:

- Strengthen your heart and lungs
- Get more oxygen into your body
- Improve mental alertness
- Elevate your mood
- Reduce your risk of heart attack and stroke
- Strengthen your bones and joints
- Improve circulation and reduce stress
- Build muscle thereby increasing your metabolism
- Decrease your appetite
- Increase calories burned
- Increase stamina, endurance and energy levels
- Increase resistance to illness and stress

Walking is the cheapest and easiest exercise. If the weather is bad you can always go to the mall or use a treadmill. On alternate days you can work with weights to build muscle and do yoga or stretching exercise to increase your flexibility. Just choose something that gets you moving.

Rebounding on a mini-trampoline is excellent for activating the lymphatic system. Movement is not only important for strength and flexibility but it also encourages our bodies to cleanse and detoxify through our elimination channels. Our bodies are mostly water. Remember, a body of water that doesn't have both incoming fresh water and an outlet stagnates and becomes a toxic cesspool.

It has to be a choice. All of it. And you have to keep making the choices over and over no matter how you feel in that moment. This applies to food, exercise, spiritual activities, everything. And every choice we make will create other choices to make. We cannot abdicate responsibility because although our choices also affect other people they mostly affect us. Priorities, degree of importance – of all the things that need to get done today what benefits you the most? You can't do all of them. Some will have to wait and they may even resolve themselves. Sometimes urgency will intervene and you have to tend to it. But every day we make hundreds of choices that determine the quality of our lives in all areas.

When you're about to blow off exercising again one more time quickly ask yourself what will be the results of either doing it or not. The pros and cons can whip through your brain quickly. Are the benefits of giving up that time in favor of something else worth it? Who's in charge? Our bodies would sit on the couch all day eating doughnuts if we'd let them. Would you let your children do that? Then why would you let yourself? Is the temporary stress relief worth the hours of guilt and remorse afterwards? I know it seems like it when it's singing its siren song. I know that in this high-stress world we live in that we get desperate for relief. We want an easy way out because everything seems so hard. Unfortunately, life is hard and there's no way around it. If there was I would have found it by now because I'm constantly looking! So since we have no choice about running this race we call life let's see how we can go for the gold.

In future chapters I will be talking about taking responsibility, keeping commitments, setting goals, planning and preparation. You will be making decisions about how you will run your race in body, soul and spirit. This is your race and you get to decide how to run it. You are not competing with anyone else. It doesn't matter what they're doing, you will decide (with God's help) what kind of race is right for you.

You will pick your training schedule and how far you go each day. You can make adjustments as you go if something is not working.

Before we go on I would like for you to do some journaling. Write about the choices you have been making and the consequences you've either enjoyed or suffered because of them.

So I just keep running my race and work on making better choices. Just for today I'm going to exercise because I know it will make me feel better. I don't have to worry about whether or not I can keep it up every day for the rest of my life. Just for today I can make some good food choices because I know that the lesser choices will give me a headache and/or cause weight gain. I will also have less energy and mental alertness. I don't have to worry about whether or not I can do this forever. Just for today I will spend time with God first thing because I want to get his guidance and protection for my day and just bask in His presence. It's just way too lonely and scary without Him. Just for today I can be pleasant to others and interested in their lives instead of going around with a frown and mentally wearing myself out by constantly tabulating my worries.

So start writing and see where it takes you. Awareness is the first step in this journey. You can't decide where to go until you know where you've been.

In addition, make an exercise choice, schedule it every day and just do it. Take into consideration your personal preferences, level of health and stamina, and time available. If you only have 15 minutes then start with that. Use every opportunity to do a little more such as taking the stairs instead of the elevator unless it's a skyscraper. Don't look for the closest parking space wherever you're going. You can park on the edge of the lot and walk to your destination. Thank God that you have body parts that you can use.

Chapter 15
De-stress Yourself

It is vitally important that you also take care of yourself in areas other than food. The amount of sleep needed varies according to individual needs but you'll know if you're shortchanging yourself. If you can barely get yourself out of bed each morning and are tired during the day then you need more hours or possibly more quality sleep. If you are too tense to go to sleep and can't get your body and brain quieted down then you need to take some measures to start gearing down before you get into bed.

I like to soak in a hot bath with Lavender essential oil in it and then read for awhile. Reading takes my mind off my worries and to-do lists. Exercise is great for de-stressing your body but you don't want to do it too close to bedtime because it can energize you. Sitting in front of the TV and stuffing food into your mouth is NOT a good option. Just think about the kinds of things that allow you to relax and write them in your daily planner. Make them a priority.

Don't let your life become too narrow with all your time taken up by work, home chores, etc. As your budget allows, plan time for massages, shopping and lunching with friends, taking a class in something you've always wanted to learn more about, meeting new people or whatever sparks your interest.

Don't neglect your spiritual life. That is where the real strength and rivers of living water come from. I had been depressed, frantic and scared lately and thought God was ignoring me. But once again I realized how important it is to seek Him instead of His blessings. When I'm in a bad place I tend to come to Him whining and complaining, totally wrapped up in my fear, worry and dread. It makes me deaf and blind and shuts me off from anything He may try to impart to me. And he does answer prayer – I've just shut down my receiver.

When I come to Him and just start praising and thanking Him then my receiver is turned on and I can sense His love and care. My mood lifts and I start getting energy and direction for the day. All of a sudden I want to get some work done, exercise, eat healthy, or do whatever needs to be done. My head is brimming with new ideas and insight. And this continues as long as I stay tuned in. By mid-afternoon if I don't get more spiritual nourishment then I start fading and going back to bad habits and negative thinking. It's like eating breakfast and nothing else the rest of the day. You get really hungry and start eating the bad stuff! So I have to remember that dwelling on negative things not only puts me in a dark mood but prevents me from receiving the good. All the ways that I've tried to escape bad feelings – eating, alcohol, shopping, reading novels, etc. – are only temporary distractions. They don't take care of the root problem which is that I let myself get disconnected from God. He didn't go away, I did, at least in my mind. And He's always there waiting for me to come back.

So build your refreshing times into your day incorporating spiritual, mental, emotional and physical. You need food and relaxation on all those levels. What have you been feeding your mind? Have you been feasting on thoughts of lack, dread, fear, and doubt or inspiration and encouragement? Whatever is going on mentally will affect your emotions. It's not your feelings that keep you from thinking positive, it's your thinking that drives your feelings. So be careful what you hear and see. Choose books, movies and TV shows that impart good things to you. We don't want to put junk food in our brain any more than we want to put junk food into our stomach. Choose your friends carefully. You're not doing either of you a favor if you hang around people who are negative and practice behaviors and attitudes that are not in line with your choices.

Make a list of pampering, stress relieving, fun, loving activities you will commit to do and put them on your calendar. They don't have to be expensive. Have you tried coloring in a coloring book since you were a child? It's very soothing.

Chapter 16
Putting It All Together

Okay, this is the hardest part – taking responsibility and keeping commitments. I know that. We have to face the fact that no one can do this for us. We have to grow up and take care of ourselves. There's no magic pill or wand that's going to cause the fat to just drop off us or make our appetites go away. We need our real appetites for survival. It's the false appetite that we have to recognize and do away with. Most of us don't know what real hunger feels like. We have lost the ability to recognize our body's signals for food, water, exercise, rest, stimulation and relaxation. We think we should always be like that famous battery bunny that just keeps going and going no matter what, constantly numbing ourselves to the cries of our body, soul and spirit. You can't keep it up forever and you'll eventually break down under it. We tend to ignore those signals also until they have reached serious proportions and are screaming at us. Then we run to whoever can give us a "fix" of some kind which is not real healing, it's just a stopgap measure and the breakdown will continue.

So STOP! Think about what you're doing to yourself and your loved ones. No one else can fix you. You are the only one who can change your situation. Gastric bypass surgery is a lousy option. I've known people who did well with it but I know of even more people who regained all the weight they lost and had new health problems to add to the old ones that prompted the surgery in the first place.

So those hungers that have nothing to do with our stomachs and food need to be addressed. Only you can discover what's missing in your life. This is not an overnight deal. It will take time and effort and continue for the rest of your life unless you just don't care about the quality of your life. People don't have quality lives because they're lucky, it's because they've worked hard at it and they never quit. I don't care how many times you fall down and have to pick yourself up again, don't ever quit. Giving up is a living death.

If you're ready to be responsible for yourself and quit whining and crying to anyone who will listen then decide what commitment you're going to make to yourself. Because you're the one you need to commit to, you're the one who will pay the biggest price and be the most disappointed if you don't keep your commitment. And lest you think I'm being hard and self-righteous I'll let you know that I'm talking to myself here too. Just having the knowledge isn't enough. You need support of others, some kind of structure and plan to enable you to keep your commitment. Find at least one person who will do this with you. Someone who will encourage, uplift and cheer you on and not nag or chastise you for stumbling. Hire God as your main coach. His only fee will be whatever you're willing to give Him. We always have free will. No one is going to make us do what's right for us – it's up to us.

Set some goals and make them realistic. Create a plan that takes into consideration what works for you personally. You're the only one that knows that based on past experience. And you'll be learning more as you go. Your daily journaling will help you know yourself and will be a good reminder when you forget that sugar makes you sick. All you have to do is look back on that day you ate it and there it is in black and white. Your plan needs to include all aspects of your life. That doesn't mean you'll never get to do anything spontaneous but leaving things up to chance is a recipe for disaster. Waiting until you're ravenous to plan your meal is not a good choice because you'll eat whatever is handy and can be quickly crammed into your mouth to stop the hunger pains. You must plan ahead. You can have occasional treats as long as you're not allergic to them or they won't cause an eating binge. Some people can handle it and some can't. Only you know you.

If you've done a lot of dieting then you already know what has worked and what hasn't. The main thing is eating whole foods and decreasing your quantity. I don't believe it's a good idea to focus on counting fat or carbohydrates exclusively. Everything should be in balance. Fruits and vegetables, preferably raw, should be the largest part of what you eat. Then legumes, starchy vegetables, meat and dairy can come after that. If you can eat whole grains without overeating them then they are fine. But if you're trying to lose weight you're better off avoiding them for now. Some people prefer to eat their biggest meal in the morning and some in the evening. I find that eating less at dinner helps me lose weight. This plan is to be created to suit your needs, not mine. So write down everything that you know about yourself and food and then your plan should start forming itself. You may need a trial and error time and your food diary will help with this. See the Recommended Food Guidelines in Chapter 19 for help.

Work with your Naturopathic Doctor or Health and Wellness Coach to determine if you need to do some cleansing and if so, what kind you should do. Your current health issues may need to be addressed by healing herbs along with the new food plan and detoxification. The healthier diet will allow your body to heal itself but it will take time. I conduct telephone consultations so you don't have to live in my area to work with me. Or you may prefer someone else. That's fine, just find a knowledgeable, reputable person to guide you.

Do not go off medications without consulting your medical doctor. Many times people have been able to gradually decrease their medications after starting their new health regime. But you will need to be monitored by your medical doctor.

If you're still having trouble with detoxification, your bowels aren't moving well or you're just feeling sluggish and toxic in general then you may need to do some colon cleansing. You don't have to do colonic hydrotherapy although I highly recommend it. You can do an herbal colon cleanse. It's just a combination of three things: herbs to cleanse and get your bowels moving, fiber for bulking the stool and acting like a broom, and bentonite clay or charcoal to soak up the toxins. It won't give you diarrhea unless you're taking too much of the herbal laxatives (such as cascara sagrada or senna) in which case you would just decrease the amount. If you're still stopped up, increase the amount. Also, taking too much fiber or bentonite clay in relation to the other elements could constipate you. It's best to buy a formula already manufactured in the proper proportions. Please email me for product recommendations.

Ongoing education is important. Take classes and read books that will increase your knowledge. Taking a raw foods preparation class with your support buddies could be lots of fun. You could get together and make large amounts and share the results. You could start a raw foods or health foods potluck in your community or just with your circle of friends. If you have a specific illness you could research more fully which foods, supplements, oils and herbs help your body in the healing process and start a support group. There's lot of possibilities and you don't ever have to be alone in this process.

If you don't live in my area and can't personally attend my classes and events then you can partake of my teleclasses and one-on-one counseling. Check my website, **http://www.DrAnnBDavis.com**, for more information.

Just know that you can succeed regardless of how many years you've been failing. All those years have taught you what doesn't work and that is valuable information. Those are the things you want to avoid at all costs. Everything in you will resist change but remember, you're the boss over your body. And with God all things are possible! We do it in His strength, not our own.

Your next assignment after creating your plan is to journal how you feel about it. Your "Chicago" is the place you most want to be. If you're not feeling a high degree of excitement, enthusiasm and optimism about going there then you must be planning someone else's "Chicago." It won't work if it's not right for you so be sure you've got that straight.

Chapter 17
Staying On Track

Okay, what's it going to take to get you to "Chicago"? What planning and preparation do you need to do?

After you've decided what your food plan will look like then you need to make some choices for your meals. Make a list of possible breakfasts, lunches, dinners and snacks. Decide what you want to eat next week and make a grocery list. I've noticed that most diet books that give you menus for a week or month have you eating something entirely different at every meal every day of the week. That's not cost efficient and it's too much work. If you're a meat eater then roast a big chicken and use the leftovers in various ways, one of my favorite being chicken-vegetable soup. It's easy, handy and low calorie. Cook a big beef roast with vegetables and use the leftovers for thin beef strips on your salad or a beef stew. Cook a big pot of beans and eat on it all week. There's nothing wrong with eating the same thing more than once. If your other family members are meat eaters then this will really help you out. Just make sure you fix lots of vegetables and salad to go with the meat. Remember, we really don't need as much meat as the meat industry would have us believe. It varies with the individual. My husband has a very fast metabolism and likes lots of meat. I don't even care if I have meat some days. I have been vegetarian at times and was quite happy.

Once you have removed sugar, flour and possibly wheat from your diet you will probably find that your hunger has significantly decreased and you're not obsessing about and craving food all the time. You may even have to remove all grains. That was true for me. I still eat starchy vegetables such as potatoes and winter squash. Sweet potatoes and butternut squash have their own sweetness and wonderful flavor and don't even need butter. With a dash of cinnamon you can pretend you're eating pumpkin pie without the crust.

Getting plenty of dark, leafy greens is very important because they are full of minerals we don't get in other foods. In addition to my green smoothies I supplement with a greens powder that contains greens, fruits, vegetables, grains, probiotics, and enzymes. You may email me for a product recommendation.

Portion control is a matter of eating when you are really and truly hungry and stopping when you're full. Full, not stuffed and bloated. If something is tempting you to keep going then just tell yourself you can have it later when you're hungry again. If you're having trouble with that in the beginning then count calories if it helps you stay in reality. Things like that are just tools to help you – they aren't meant to run your life. Use smaller plates and serve yourself half of what you usually eat and then give your stomach time to decide if that was enough. If it wasn't then have a little more. Remember, we live in America where food is plentiful. We don't have to hoard it in our bodies. It's easy to obtain more.

Create a safety net with preparation and planning. It's not a suit of armor in which you'll be trapped if you make flexibility and choices a part of it. But having that plan in place keeps you from going off the rails.

After your menus and shopping list are done then you need to make a list of your daily chores where food is concerned. Some produce can be washed and made ready when you get home from shopping, like lettuce. Others may need to wait until you're ready for them because they wouldn't keep as well. Your daily chore list is to make sure you have everything ready that you need so you don't get home from work starving and have everything either in the freezer or needing a lot of prep work. Keep it simple. This is not a time for gourmet recipes. You don't want to get bored with your food but you don't want to be spending a lot of time in the kitchen either or you'll feel like a galley slave.

Take the time to go through your kitchen and throw away all the refined, processed junk and make room for the good stuff you're going to buy. Clean out your kitchen and rearrange it so that it's more handy to work in.

In addition to your daily food chores you'll need a schedule for exercise, prayer, meditation, etc. If all this seems like a lot of work, it is! But that's what successful people do – they plan their work and work their plan. If your slipshod methods were working you wouldn't be reading this book. It's just a matter of how badly you want to get to "Chicago." There is no magic bullet. If you're not naturally organized, then this is the time to learn how.

It takes time to get your mind and mouth renewed but it can be done. It takes diligence and perseverance. You may have to give up a little sleep time or arrange for your spouse to be with your children so you can have some quiet time. If you've been saying negative things about yourself and your situation then that has to change. What you say is what you get. You do not want to create negative energy around yourself. It's too easy to go into a downward spiral once you start thinking and speaking negative.

I realize that most people have a lot of obligations (work, spouse, children, etc.) that they can't just ignore while they work on themselves. It all has to be managed. But how can you be the best you can be for anyone else if you're overwhelmed, depressed, tired, sick and defeated? You may have to have a talk with your family about how you need to take care of yourself. Let them know the things that you need to do and why. Of course, showing them how it will benefit them also will get a better buy-in from them. You probably can't put your whole family on your food plan because they either don't need it or are not willing. Everyone needs to eat more healthy foods but may need more calories. My husband couldn't survive on the amount of calories that are right for me. So I cook some things for him that I don't eat myself. He understands how I need to have some types of food banned from the house. Fortunately, some of the things he likes are not a temptation for me. You know your family better than anyone. How can you negotiate with them so that you can get the support you need to make these changes? If you've ever taken an airplane trip you'll know that the flight attendants always tell you to put your oxygen mask on before you put it on your child because you're not any use to them dead. The same principle applies here. This is one of those times when you need to put yourself and your health first and everyone will reap the benefits. If they are willing to try some of your healthier foods then eventually you may be able to prepare the same foods for everyone. But you can't force it on them. They'll be impressed when they start to see positive changes in you.

Chapter 18
Plug Into the Power

I've struggled my entire life with feelings of powerlessness, futility, negativity, despair, hopelessness, not being good enough, on and on. I was never taught to think positive about anything or to value myself. I'm not blaming my parents. They were just passing on what they were taught. We have so much more knowledge and help available to us now then we ever had before but there are still many people who never utilize it. Having it in your head is not useful if you don't understand it in your heart.

As I continued in my studies of God, abundance, prosperity, health and my purpose in life I discovered that my belief system was my biggest problem. I had a hard time really believing that God wanted to bless me and be a part of my everyday life. I could not bring myself to trust Him. I thought if I read enough books and studied enough I could figure it all out, do it right and be safe. I analyzed myself into paralysis and became more and more fearful of doing anything. I just knew I'd mess it up. I wasn't willing to step out in faith because I wanted to know the whole plan ahead of time.

Years ago I got the inner knowing that inside of me are all the answers I would ever need. I didn't understand it at the time and always looked to other people for my answers. But their answers weren't my answers so that didn't always work out. Plus people usually have their own agenda when they give you an answer or it may just be what worked for them. The more I depended upon others to guide me the more powerless I felt.

But in the past couple of years I've been realizing that I'm not ever going to get all the answers ahead of time. I only get them as I need them. And there are spiritual laws that I had been ignorant of. "You have not because you ask not" and

"Ask, believing that you receive, and you will have it." I had read them many times in the Bible but didn't understand or believe them. It has always been difficult for me to ask anyone for help. I just assumed the answer would be "no." And I never believed that I was good enough to receive anything good.

As I've continued to study and seek God my belief level has risen tremendously. I started noticing more and more that I was asking and getting answers. All the things I had obsessed about trying to make happen, if I just asked for what I needed and then let it go, eventually happened. Not always exactly when and how I thought it should but the answers were always on time and just what I needed.

So I don't need to have personal power. My power comes from believing and trusting in God and letting Him live through me. I am a unique manifestation of Him because I'm different from everyone else. No, I'm not perfect and sometimes I don't reflect His presence but that's only because I've stopped the flow somehow. It's just a basic 'On/Off' situation and we get to control the switch. The more I choose 'On' the better my life flows. When I choose 'Off' I end up in the ditch.

Trying to do it by yourself is just too hard so why not take this journey with the One who loves you best?

Chapter 19
Recommended Food Guidelines

- 75% fruits and vegetables, 75% of them raw, 25% can be baked or steamed vegetables.

- 25% remaining for meat, nuts, seeds, grains, legumes, oils.

- All fruits and vegetables allowed but don't go overboard on fruit. Use dark leafy greens, not iceberg lettuce.

- Cooked vegetables can include sweet potatoes and winter squash as well as all the low starch vegetables.

- Meat should be organic or free range. Fish should be wild caught, not farm raised. Focus on mostly fish.

- Dairy should be only organic, unsweetened, cultured products such as yogurt and kefir in small quantities. No milk. Some people need to eliminate dairy entirely.

- Oils include olive, flax, coconut.

- Grains are whole grains or sprouted grains only. No flour products. Examples are buckwheat, millet, quinoa, and oats. Bread should be sprouted grain only such as Ezekiel 4:9 by Food for Life. They also make sprouted grain tortillas.

- Pasta is never a good choice whatever it's made of but you can bake spaghetti squash and it spoons up in beautiful strands just like pasta. It's delicious with a marinara sauce on it.

- Beans and peas can be part of the cooked portion or sprouted for salad.

- Eggs are okay every way but fried.

- Nuts and seeds, raw, in moderation (no peanuts).

- Raw cultured vegetables such as sauerkraut or kimchee (an Oriental dish).

- One quart of green smoothie a day or more.

- Stevia is the best choice for sweetener. NuNaturals brand is best. No sugar or artificial sweetener.

- Water – drink half your weight in ounces of water daily.

- **AVOID** sugar, flour products, preservatives, additives, chemicals, MSG, caffeine, excessive salt, chips, fried foods, artificial sweeteners, and food dyes.

Menu Suggestions

I believe in keeping it simple because I don't like to prepare food and most of us are too busy to spend much time in the kitchen anyway. If you like to try out recipes then check out the list of raw food websites I've included in the book. I've listed the suggestions in order of preference for this program. Some choices are about equal so don't over-analyze!

Breakfast

- Green smoothie.
- Just fruit.
- Fruit and raw granola.
- Fruit and yogurt.
- Eggs and sprouted grain toast. Add veggies to scrambled eggs.
- Oatmeal with 1-2 tsp. of nut butter stirred in or raw nuts or seeds and fruit.

Lunch and Dinner – always have a salad with your meal

- Green smoothie.
- Green salad with variety of vegetables and homemade raw dressing.
- Salad with grilled meat on it, lots of different veggies, beans, etc. Watch out for bottled dressings with sugar and chemicals in them. Just make your own basic vinaigrette.
- Lettuce wraps.
- Wraps using sprouted grain tortillas. Just add meat and lots of veggies and roll up.
- Soups and stews.
- Grilled or baked meat/fish with big salad and potatoes, winter squash, or other veg.
- Baked potato with veggies on top.
- Spaghetti and sauce (with or without meat) using baked spaghetti squash instead of pasta. Try using ground turkey or chicken instead of ground beef.

- Chili using lots of beans and diced veggies in it such as bell peppers, celery, carrots. You can also use ground chicken or turkey instead of beef.

Snacks

- Fresh vegetable juice.
- Fruit.
- Raw veggies.
- Hummus with veggies.
- Nuts – just a few.

Dessert

- Fruit. Also, can add yogurt or yogurt cheese and a few nuts.

Chapter 20
Getting Started

To make the green smoothie, put 2 cups of water in your blender, add two large handfuls of greens such as organic baby spinach, and 2 cups of fruit. Some of the fruit can be frozen. Experiment with different kinds to see which ones you like. The spinach is mild and you will not taste it. If you use other greens that are stronger, add a lemon or lime to the smoothie and it will cut the strong taste. You can add ice if you like it real cold and aren't using frozen fruit and a little stevia if you like it sweeter. Blend until smooth and drink slowly. If you get full before you finish it just save the remainder in the refrigerator for later. If you desire, you can have just green smoothies for days or even weeks as a cleansing protocol. As long as you vary the fruits and vegetables you will get a balanced diet. This is much easier than trying to do a juice or water fast and much safer.

If you experience detox symptoms at any time such as headache, achy body, nausea, excessive mucus discharge, insomnia, then cut back on the amount of raw food you're eating until it passes then resume. It is helpful to get an IonCleanse footbath at this time to help pull out toxins. You could also take an Epsom salt bath. If you are constipated then colon hydrotherapy or an enema is helpful. You can also take magnesium to help hydrate the bowel and/or an herbal laxative like cascara sagrada to promote peristalsis. Start with a small amount and increase until you get the results you desire. You'll know you're using too much if you get diarrhea. Even better is doing a colon cleanse program.

I have created the **Rawesome Living System** which combines the healthy diet and lifestyle tips outlined in this book along with some of the supplements mentioned. You

may contact me about this program and receive a free
30 minute consultation.

If you have any questions or concerns not answered here then
please email me at **rawesomeliving@yahoo.com**.

Appendix A

My favorite supplements come from a couple of different companies. It's best if you email me for more detailed information about the products and assistance with ordering. That way I can help you choose the products that are best suited for you.

Please email me at **rawesomeliving@yahoo.com** if you have questions about anything I've mentioned in this book. You can also go to my website at **http://www.DrAnnBDavis.com** to learn more about my offerings.

Appendix B

The raw food recipe book that I recommend for beginners is *Raw Food Made Easy* by Jennifer Cornbleet.

For learning more about green smoothies, I highly recommend Victoria Boutenko's book *Green for Life*. The Boutenko family has a fascinating story and other books that are all great. You can visit their website at **http://www.rawfamily.com**.

There are also a lot of videos on **YouTube** that show you how to prepare raw food and green smoothies plus there are many websites out there with lots of information and recipes. Just do a search on "raw food" or "green smoothies".

A website with loads of raw food education and recipes, and reasonably priced appliances is **http://www.living-foods.com**. There are so many great raw food websites out there. Just be aware that there are a lot of conflicting opinions and some of them are pretty radical.

Another favorite is **Simply Salads** by Jennifer Chandler. It has a picture for every recipe (a feature I love) and there is such a variety you can make a different one every day for weeks. They are simple, quick and easy and use pre-washed greens and a few other ingredients. Some of the recipes have meat or fish to go with them.

You should be able to find all of these on **http://www.amazon.com**.

www.ingramcontent.com/pod-product-compliance
Lightning Source LLC
Chambersburg PA
CBHW060217290526
45789CB00003B/1302